The Carbogenic Body Type

Representing one of the 22 Body Types first described by Victor Rocine around 1900

The Hugh Jackman, Annette Benning Celebrity Body Type

For Kaye,
there at the beginning with Doc Severn,
and for Liberty,
continuing the holistic healing journey…

Disclaimer

The information in this book is for educational purposes only and is not a substitute for medication, diets, or other medical care. The diets do not treat diseases or medical conditions, and are an adjunct to your orthodox health care.

The author and publisher accept no responsibility for any misuse of the information within. If you have any physical problem, food allergy, emotional disorder, or disease, common sense dictates that you consult with a physician before changing your diet, taking nutritional supplements, or following the advice given here.

———

About the Author

Educated in New Zealand and in the U.S.A., Dr. Stenbeck attained B.Sc. (NZ), M.S., and D.C. degrees. His holistic healing methods have been profiled in magazines (Esquire, McLean's, Playgirl, the Atlanta Constitution), and on TV in the USA and in Canada. He was the main contributor to the Warner Book, _The Eye/Body Connection_ by Jessica Maxwell that focused on the holistic healing relationships between the iris structure and organ genetics.

In the 1970-80's he was elected Fellow, Royal Society of Health, London; Fellow, American Association of Chemists; Member, American Association of Clinical Chemists; and Affiliate, Royal Society of Medicine, London. He studied naturopathy and Body Types with Dr. Bernard Jensen and Dr. Clifford Severn, and has practiced in medical partnerships where patients received the joint benefits of medica

He is a member of Self-Realization Fellowship. To receive advice on any health issue from a holistic viewpoint, or to receive help with your body type, see his web site: *DrStenbeck.net*

———

Contents

* * *

The Carbogenic Body Type (and Food Guide)   1

* * *

The 22 Body Types: Celebrity Examples

This Booklet contains the **Carbogenic** *type. [See* <u>*The 22 Unique Body Types*</u> *for all type descriptions.]*

Thin Types

Atrophic   *Woody Allen / Audrey Hepburn*
               Stan Laurel / Calista Flockheart

Exesthesic   *Cher / Sarah Jessica Parker*
               (Female type only)

Marasmic   *President Obama / Princess Diana*
               James Stewart / Kate Blanchard

Neurogenic   *J.K. Simmons / Joan Rivers*
               Jon Cryer / Marin Hinle

Pathoferic   *(No celebrity males)*
               Blythe Danner / Gwyneth Paltrow

Sillevitic   *David Bowie / Shirley MacLaine*
               Rod Stewart / Carol Channing

Muscle Types

Calciferic   *Michael Jordan / Angelica Huston*
Abraham Lincoln / Grace Jones

Carbogenic   *George Clooney / Lady Gaga*
Pres. Donald Trump / Meg Ryan

Desmogenic   *Marlon Brando / Loni Anderson*
Daniel Craig / Tina Turner

Eldic   *Ross Perot / Hillary Clinton*
Peter Falk / Sigourney Weaver

Myogenic   *Pres. Bill Clinton / Sharon Stone*
Pres. John Kennedy / Julia Roberts

Medeic   *Gary Oldman / Madonna*
John Hurt / Marlene Deitrich

Nervimotive   *Frank Sinatra / Elizabeth Taylor*

Nitropheric   *Ben Affleck / Ava Gardner*
Kirk Douglas / Kate Winslet

Pallinomic   *President Lyndon Johnson /*
Attorney General Janet Reno /
Bill O'Reilly (Fox) / Jane Russell

Fat Types

Barotic   *Robin Williams / 'Mrs.Doubtfire'*
                     Elton John / William Conrad

Carboferic   *Bill Murray / Roseanne*
                     Billy Gardell / Melissa McCarthy

Hydripheric   *John Goodman / Shelly Winters*
                     Wayne Knight / Jennifer Holliday

Isogenic   *Einstein / Oprah Winfrey*
                     Phillip S .Hoffman / Queen Victoria

Lipopheric   *Rush Limbaugh / Rosie O'Donnell*
                     Chris Christie / Camryn Manheim

Oxypheric   *Winston Churchill / Orsen Welles*
                     Ella Fitzgerald / Gerry Spence

Pargenic   *President Richard Nixon /*
                     Katey Segal
                     Ron Perlman / Kirstey Alley

<u>*Succinct Quote on Human Types*</u>

From Victor Rocine, who first described discrete body types around 1900.

"A type is an order of people that differentiates and distinguishes itself by a general and similar form, brain-formation, chemistry, structure, build, immunity, tendencies, predisposition, resemblance, skin-pigment, and type characteristics based on observation and analogy.

"Or, in other words, people of a given type are similar physically and like-minded as if they were brothers and sisters—that is what type means.

"Everything in nature is made according to plan. Man only discovers that plan and gives it a name. The zoologist has not made the animals—he has only described the plan adopted by the wonderful Creator, and named the classes, sub-classes, etc.

"How important type research will be to humanity, time alone will make known."

———

Prologue

The esteemed scientist J. J. Berzelius, discoverer of several chemical elements, inspired Victor Rocine to research body types and to investigate the correlation between types and their diseases. Around 1890-1910, Rocine privately published his original findings on the mineral basis of different body types, and this present book exists because of his brilliant insights.

For many years, I studied with Dr. Clifford Severn who had been a personal student of Victor Rocine on body types, naturopathy, herbology, iris analysis, diet, and nutritional healing methods. He had a successful career as a lecturer and healer, and was one of those rare athletes with complete muscle control over his body. I saw him under a spotlight at 85 years of age, contracting and rippling every individual muscle in his perfectly developed body. Field-Marshal Jan Smuts, the WWII South African Prime Minister, devoted a full chapter of his autobiography to how Severn's healing methods had saved his life. In the 1950's, *Life* magazine did a four-page spread on Severn and his family. Fame he had.

Another Rocine student I studied with, Dr. Bernard Jensen wrote of Rocine's body type research and nutritional methods in his privately published book *The Chemistry of Man*.

This book is deeply rooted in Rocine's original work, and with that of Herbert Shelton, M.D., Ph.D. (at Harvard University in the 1930's). I integrated their research with newer dietary and nervous system data along with celebrity examples of each type, hopefully, making this material easier to digest and more entertaining for the reader.

Gayelord Hauser, another Rocine student I knew, was a celebrated health book author. He wrote a popular book on Rocine's types in the 1940's, *Types and Temperaments;* reputedly, he also introduced yogurt to the western world.

This book exists because of Rocine's creative brilliance and original discoveries in natural healing.

► *Rocine: "The soul creates the body type."*

Rocine taught that the soul chooses a body type and brain to live in, thus presenting different experiences and life lessons to master. Why were *you* born the way you are?

That is something to think about, especially if it is true! What would your soul purpose be to live in a particular body type. I provide some thoughts on this issue in each type description and try to assess from my experience with your type the particular lessons of life presented therein.

Rocine was as brilliant in his way as an Abraham Lincoln, Michael Jordan, Michael Phelps, or Tony Robbins—all *calciferic* types —rare, leaders, innovative, brilliant, and highly intelligent in their different fields of endeavor.

Celebrity examples exist for most types, not a duplicate of you, but someone who has your essence in their body-mind individuality. Knowing your type allows you to become a better you! The celebrity examples provide further help in identifying your body type.

▶ *Rocine's classic findings are the backbone of this book. Integrated with Sheldon's research and with other dietary and food issues including mental, emotional, and spiritual attributes,*

Many people take nutritional supplements and try different diets without a doctor's advice. If this is your choice, use common sense, listen to body responses, and discontinue any allergic reactions to foods or nutritional substances.

———

The Carbogenic
Body Type

* * *

*"You may also have a physical or psychological
feature not representative of your type such as
height, weight, appearance, talent, weakness,
strength, etc., due to biochemical errors,
environmental influences, racial or cultural
differences, and congenital or genetic issues.
Nevertheless, the type identification in the
average person is usually clear."*

— *Victor Rocine*

Carbogenic Type Celebrity Examples

If you think this is your type, be sure to look at **on-line photographs** *of these examples. Look for general similarities to yourself. Note that sub-types cause the differences in appearance between members of the same type. There are many good examples listed of this frequently found type.*

———

GOVERNMENT

President Donald Trump*
President Jimmy Carter
President George W. Bush
Pres. Candidate Senator Lieberman
VP Hubert Humphrey
Pres. Candidate Senator Ted Cruz
Prime Minister Tony Blair
George Stephanopoulos (Pres. Clinton
    advisor; commentator)

———

* President Trump's physical appearance differs from most other examples because of his pallinomc subtype, which has a larger body and often a more abrasive personality; checkout earlier photos of him up to his thirties, where he shows the more classical carbogenic type appearance.

ACTORS (many Oscars)

Robert Downey, Jr.

George Clooney	William DeVane
Hugh Grant	Bruce Willis
John Travolta	Alec Baldwin
Andy Garcia	Josh Dallas
David Bernie	Alan Alda
Joe Mantegna	Peter Sellers
Dennis Hopper	Gary Sinese
Gene Kelly	Steve Martin
Richard Dryfuss	Tony Curtis
Robert Conrad	Dudley Moore
William Baldwin	Hugh Jackman
John Mills	Ron Silver
Jay Thomas	Roy Rogers
Dick Powell	Robert Taylor
Robert Blake	Ted Dansen
Ben Gazzara	Jude Law
Audie Murphy	Joe Mortaegna
Jim Parsons	Jim Carey
Richard Simmons	Eric Estrada
Marv Albert	Dick Clark
Tim Allen	Tom Brokaw
John Slattery	Michael Sheen
Tom Selleck	Dean Martin
Mike Farrell	Pierce Brosnan
Steve Martin	

Annette Benning	Liza Minelli
Drew Barrymore	Bonnie Bedelia
Dolly Parton	Goldie Hawn

Charlene Tilton	Judy Garland
Jeanie Garth	Nancy Allen
Sally Field	Betty Grable
Bernadette Peters	Jean Harlow
Shelly Fabre	Paris Hilton
Debbie Reynolds	Jerry Hall
Mariette Hartley	Sarah Palin
Meg Ryan	Christina Applegate

April Bowlby (Kandi, *"Two and Half Men"*)

SPORTS

Muhammad Ali	Andy Murray
Novak Djokovic	Oscar de la Hoya

Lionel Messi (soccer)

Jackie Robinson (Many pro-athletes, Grand Prix drivers)

ARTS/OTHER

Anderson Cooper

Anthony Bourdain (CNN)

Shepard Smith (Fox)

Miles Davis	Julian Assange
Simon Cowell	Michael Feinstein
Hugh Heffner	Richard Branson
Steve Jobs	Colonel Oliver North
Steven Spielberg	George Lucas
Paul Simon	Joel Osteen
Elvis	Richard Benjamin
Robert Goulet	Paul McCartney
Bobby Darin	Justin Bieber

Duke Ellingon   Louis Armstrong
Rudy Valli   Andre Previn
Mark Fuhrman   Chef Ramsay

Bernadette Peters Paula Abdul
Mariah Carey   Stevie Nicks
Lady Gaga
Laura Logan ("60 Minutes")

[Note: I personally knew eight of the above celebrities, and many others in everyday life, which contributed much to my understanding of the type.]

You already know something about this type from their public persona and appearance, whether from seeing them yourself or from the celebrity examples. Blend such insights with the type descriptions and the types of your family and friends to discern their presence in your midst!

Read the types and if still confused you may choose to use the personal request for type identification from the Appendix or from my web site: *DrStenbeck.net*

———

▶ *My celebrity type identifications, mostly from photos and movies, **cannot** be 100% accurate, and I assess my typing at about 80% accurate.*

Carbogenic Type Questionnaire

These questions describe the generic type, and not specifically you! If any question ever applied to you, then choose the True answer!

For Question 1 only:

A = True	*B = Maybe*	*C = Untrue*
15 points	*7 points*	*1 point*

1. Physically identify with celebrity example____

Then…

A = True	*B = Maybe*	*C = Untrue*
5 points	*3 points*	*1 point*

---

2. Height is close to:
   Males: 5'2-6'4   Females: 5'0-5'8   ____
3. Usual weight is close to:
   Males: 150-230   Females: 110–150   ____
4. Both sexes highly sensual   ____
5. Muscles are medium-sized or large,
   Potential high strength   ____
6. Somewhat sensitive, nervous persona   ____
7. Rectangular forehead   ____
8. Hair growth plentiful throughout life
   (unless a balding sub-type is present)   ____
9. Nose often smaller than average,
   may heave pinched nostrils   ____

10. Face has small cheekbones, may have cheek indentations _____
11. Strong ego, egocentric (some males) _____
12. Skin lovely and white when young _____
13. Teeth average-sized, white _____
14. Crave money, comfort _____
15. Fearful, anxious, concerned _____
16. Many workaholics, or may be lazy _____
17. Charming, sympathetic, friendly _____
18. A highly developed sense of humor _____
19. Hard-working, serious work ethic _____
20. Gourmet tastes are common _____
21. Able to entertain or talk for hours _____
22. Have a moderate or strong sex drive _____
23. Males hairy chest; bust medium-large (unless lost through weight loss) _____
24. Loving, sympathetic, friendly _____
25. Some may drink or use drugs _____
26. Voice soft, kind, interested _____
27. Use gentle persuasion, peaceful talk _____
28. Many males prematurely grey by 25-30 _____
29. Fall in love easily; affectionate lovers _____
30. Males have a beard-line _____
31. Often hypoglycemic from sugars, cookies, ice cream, etc. _____
32. Inclined to metaphysics, conspiracy theories, supernatural _____
33. Naturally assertive or aggressive _____
34. Some have cravings or addictions _____
35. Acting-musical talents common:, singing, performing, writing, etc. _____

36. Easily become sick from excessive
    sugars and starches   _____
37. May believe can do things better
    than other people   _____
38. Some are co-dependent or controlling
    in relationships   _____
39. Tend to a high level of jealousy   _____
40. May hold grudges   _____
41. Have a seductive energy   _____
42. May be moody if don't get own way   _____
43. Self-control may be weak   _____
44. Inclined to be secretive   _____
45. Are particularly loving to those who
    do much for them   _____
46. Usually polite and respectful   _____
47. May give up too easily on a project   _____
48. Some are arrogant (particularly males) _____
49. Some are lazy and passive   _____
50. Inclined to procrastinating   _____
51. Enjoy communicating with others   _____
52. Usually pretty, beautiful, or handsome _____
53. Are extremely confident   _____
54. Good sports ability (mostly males)   _____
55. Desire independence   _____
56. Some may easily become grouchy   _____
57. If provoked, particularly males will
    'fight to the death'   _____

Scoring

For question #1:
A response: give 15 points   = _____

B response: give 7 points   = _____

C response: give 1 points   = _____

For questions #2—57:
A response: give 5 points   = _____

B response: give 3 points   = _____

C response: give 1 point   = _____

Total of the above points   = _____

Interpretation
149—275: PROBABLY Carbogenic type

74—148: POSSIBLY Carbogenic type

<74: NOT Carbogenic type

The Carbogenic Type

"Carbogenic refers to your overactive starch and carbohydrate metabolism. You may excessively absorb food carbon, which undermines your health. You are often deficient in the essential healing element, calcium."

The *carbogenic* type is medium-sized and strong with attractive males and lovely or beautiful females. You show a combination of strength, charm, intelligence, and an honest work ethic. You achieve success through self-activation, and employers appreciate your hard work. Immortalized in World War II, Betty Grable was the Gi pin-up poster-girl. Your type proliferates in Asian, Mediterranean, Middle-Eastern, and Latin countries (and to a lesser degree in the USA).

▶ *Both sexes cause hearts to flutter because of their attractiveness, beauty, sensuality, honesty, and a friendly smile and deportment. You often have a lovely or handsome face, and a shapely body.*

You have excellent social skills, and high intelligence. You accomplish much in acting, singing, dancing, behind the camera work, etc., as with Dolly Parton, Drew Barrymore, George Clooney, Alec Baldwin, Steven Spielberg, and George Lucas. Love may cause suffering in younger females because of low self-esteem or co-dependency: you may attract abusive males (and vise versa). Some may settle for too little in life. You have strong love and sensual instincts (with many playboys being of this type).

You have a highly developed sense of humor, some being able to entertain people for hours with jokes and stories. The males are attractive, handsome, muscled, often having a hairy chest and back, and may be very strong. You tend to have a beard-line and look like you need a shave (like the *pargenic*). Other types may also have body hair, particularly the *nervimotive and pargenic* (with whom you may be confused), whereas the *nitropheric* and *medeic* men mostly have little or no body hair. You know you look good, are winners, and usually succeed in the world.

Physical Similarity to Other Types

The lean *nervimotive* (Frank Sinatra, Lesley Ann Warren) is somewhat similar and has a nervous persona.

The *neurogenic* type (Martin Short, Jane Seymour) is friendly, pretty, nervous, and talkative.

The *neurogenic* is often the sub-type of the *carbogenic*.

––––––

Average Height and Weight

Males:	5'2-6'4	150-230 pounds
Females:	5'0-5'8	110-150 pounds

––––––

Carbogenic Type Description

The type description represents how you appear in everyday society. You may have a sub-type that alters parts of this description.

Think of the celebrity examples as you read the descriptions. A small percentage of the males are quite short as in Michael J. Fox. *Carbogenics* like Judy Garland and her daughter Liza Minelli have fat sub-types *(carboferic)* that necessarily makes fat accumulation a problem. You are attractive, or beautiful, and have harmonious figures when young; you look fit and healthy, and the males are often very strong.

Head — You have a somewhat oval and smooth head on frontal view; the forehead is medium-sized and rectangular.

Hair — Hair growth is plentiful, lovely, and abundant, with most of you maintaining a full head of hair throughout life; males are usually grey or white by age 30. Numerous males are attracted to wearing a pony-tail. Fair and brown shades predominate in females, with dark brown and black shades in the males.

Eyes — Your eye color is usually blue, light brown or hazel, with a sincere and honest expression.

Ears — Normal-sized ears set close to the head are typical.

Nose — The nose is usually smaller than average, with pinched nostrils.

Face — You have subtle cheekbones without cheek indentations. Some of you have a relatively short distance between the eyes and mouth; your face usually ages gracefully.

Mouth and Lips — The lips are full, affectionate, attractive, and sensuous; a normal-sized and shaped mouth is usual. Your voice is soft, kind, low-pitched, sympathetic, concerned, and interested.

Teeth —You have average-sized, white, strong attractive teeth (if not calcium deficient).

Skin — Your skin is lovely and white-tinted when young; acne may occur if you are unhealthy.

Neck —A muscular and strong neck is usual.

Muscles —Your muscles are medium-sized or larger, and of moderate to high strength with many professional athletes being of this type, as in boxing, baseball, soccer, tennis, etc. You are able to build superb muscle definition, like Hugh Jackman, in 'X Men'. (Most heavyweight boxers are *desmogenic.*)

▶ *I have known several males who said that if forced to fight, they would go to their death before going down. You are great infantry soldiers like the actor and most highly decorated US soldier of WWII, Audie Murphy.*

Chest — The males often have a hairy chest (and upper torso) while some have less hair growth (due to the sub-type). The females have a medium or large bust, which may be easily lost following quick weight-loss diets.

Back and Shoulders — These areas are moderately strong.

Hips and Abdomen — Your hips and abdomen are medium-sized.

Arms and Legs —There is a harmonious and handsome shape to the extremities. Your hands and feet are often small with tapering fingers.

Joints — Strong bones, joints, and tendons are common.

———

Carbogenic Personality Traits

If you are this Muscle type many, but not all, of the following characteristics are present—you may have overcome or moderated the negatives, but recognize that you once had several of them.

You may have any of the following traits:

- An efficient and tenacious mind
- Assertive or aggressive (ready to do battle)
- Are highly sociable; respect mental superiors

- Are honest workers with a serious work ethic
- Many are well suited for the police or military
- May be nervous, often fearful (but not neurotic)
- Some are inclined to metaphysics, conspiracies
- High courage, bravery; usually are 'adrenalin junkies'
- Usually polite, diplomatic, and respectful
- Attitude of *supreme* self-confidence, friendliness
- Strongly desire a comfortable life, independence
- Generally a highly developed sense of h-umor (many comedians)
- Have acting or musical sense: whether listening, playing, singing, performing, directing, or writing (e.g., Hugh Jackman)
- Have a loving, sympathetic, congenial, honest, and friendly nature; some males may be brusque, arrogant, "macho" and risk takers
- May crave sweets, sugars, cookies, ice cream, etc., more than most types, and become sick from over-eating them.

▶ *Rocine: "You lead and rule by gentle persuasion, peace, quiet, and persuasive talking,"*
Excellent examples are Presidents Carter, George Bush Jr., Senator Lieberman, British Prime Minister Tony Blair.

———

Potential Challenges

You may have evolved from, or not experienced these common faults, so do not dwell on them.

▶ *I have known some males who would become drunk and insist on driving: alcohol and drugs may discard reason and common sense. Younger females may wake up in someone's bed and not know how they got there!*

- Some feel victimized by life
- Do not like displeasing others
- Some are lazy, weak will-power
- Strongly dislike fumes and noise
- Are easily hurt if goals are not met
- Males may be macho and demanding
- Mat hold grudges, be secretive, jealous
- May whine, complain, worry about trivia
- Females, when young, may be submissive

- Tend to be grouchy, moody if crossed
- Males are often ego-centric, controlling
- May give up too easily and feel that all is lost
- Cravings common to alcohol, nicotine (males)
- Sensual energy when young (particularly males)
- Some cannot stop talking (and are not good listeners)
- Some males have low self-control around sex, alcohol, drugs
- Some are arrogant (particularly males) from very high self-confidence
- Able to sell anything to anybody; some males are superb 'con-men' who make great sales-persons due to excessive self-confidence

―――――

Carbogenic Stress Management

Your mental stress prevention is vulnerable, and you may internalize thinking stress and worries into your stomach, adrenals, and immune system. Emotional stress prevention is variable, and you may need re-programming of negative emotions.

[If needing help managing these stresses, see my prior books.]

———

Love

You appreciate a mate who is gentle, honest, respectful, and spiritual. You are physically affectionate and usually attracted to the *calciferic, eldic, myogenic, marasmic, neurogenic, nervimotive, nitropheric, and pathoferic* types. There is generally a moderate to strong sex drive, some males desiring sex several times daily.

———

Talents and Vocations

I have known or observed your type in many actors, chefs, doctors, artists, secretaries, real estate, entrepreneurial millionaires, professional athletes, advertising persons, racing car drivers, jet fighter and airline pilots. You are often adrenalin junkies.

Abilities - *Industry, arts, decorating, buying, marketing, negotiating*

You often work in restaurant and other small businesses. President Carter, a peacemaker, is gentle, persuasive, trusted, and honest. Usually, you find a way to succeed. The type information cannot predict what or who you will become, but you are capable of bringing a creative excellence or brilliance to whatever you do in life.

Inabilities - *Executives, science*

You have medium-executive ability and work better serving others.

————

Health Problems

▶ *Rocine found that eating daily calcium and dairy foods are keys to your healing. Eating them excessively enhances aging diseases!*

When sick, you may experience any of the following health problems:

Cardio-vascular — A high cholesterol or triglycerides is commonly found.

Diabetes — Diabetes may be in your family history: the over-eating of simple sugars and carbohydrates threatens your health.

Lungs — The lungs are vulnerable to infection.
Hypoglycemia — This is common with fatigue, sugar cravings, headaches, depression, and back pain (from sugar and a bad diet).

Stomach Problems — You readily internalize mental stress and anxieties into your stomach, causing ulcers, etc.

———

Carbogenic Acid/Alkaline Factor

For your health and healing, the genetics of your autonomic nervous system predispose you to needing a specific ratio of food acidity to alkalinity. You are born with an *alkaline* constitution, which means you need a predominantly **acid-ash** food intake for acid/alkaline balance. (Ash refers to the minerals left in your body after metabolizing foods.) Your nervous system genetics are *parasympathetic* dominant, and theoretically, you need about 70% acid-ash foods (proteins, carbo-hydrates) in your diet, but…

For your healing, if in ill health or after about age 40-45, you need to aim for this approximate ratio of food selections:
  50% Proteins, carbohydrates
  50% Fruits, salads, vegetables

▶ *Approximate your food ratios. On any particular day, it does not matter if one meal is mostly alkaline and another mostly acid—just try to balance it out for the day! If you make a mistake, try again tomorrow. It is a subjective call that you make, as what you do over weeks and months makes the difference to your health.*

———

The Carbogenic Spiritual Factor

Skip this paragraph if uninterested in a philosophical perspective on your type!

▶ *Rocine: "The soul chooses the body type."*

If as souls, we choose the brain and body type to spend a lifetime in, it could be to learn certain spiritual lessons related to perfecting ourselves, and our humanity, in God's eyes. What lessons does the type bring you? Only you can really decide what those lessons are. You know your weaknesses, faults, and behaviors towards others. You know things about yourself that Victor Rocine could never get from his research subjects when he first wrote about types. So search your mind for the answers.

Each discrete type has challenges of life lessons, spiritual goals, etc., and some of yours may be:

Faith — Most often, your faith is from what you see and touch. Having faith in a higher power is difficult for you. You need to seek, find and enhance your God relationship.

Alcohol or Drugs — Some of you are vulnerable to addiction and need therapy, but denial is common (in both sexes).

Ego — Many males, particularly, tend to be ego-centric and may have macho behavior. You need psychological help with this (although few will admit it)!

Co-dependent — May have difficulty forming de-voted loving relationships; young females of this type may be submissive to macho men, while the *carbogenic* males tend to be dominating. Realize that your attractiveness, beauty, and sensuality get in the way of others appreciating you for your considerable intelligence and brain power. A *supreme* self-confidence, particularly in males, may attract co-dependent women.

————

A Carbogenic Story…

Julie, age 24, 5'4, shapely and pretty, complained of fatigue, mood swings, depression, and sugar craving; her medical exams were negative. I found a calcium deficiency and increased her calcium food intake with kelp, parsley, Swiss and cheddar cheese, turnip greens, Brewer's yeast, almonds, and corn tortillas.

Along with her calcium need, which was very important for her type and healing, she needed to minimize simple sugars and carbon foods: carbohydrates, starches, grains, breads, and white sugar foods. Removing these substances from the diet was essential to her health.

Julie followed the dietary recommendations, took 1,500 mg/day of supplemental calcium, and her low blood sugar symptoms resolved completely. Her problem was subclinical, not a disease.

Note - The following recommendations are for the generic type. Additionally, you may need from a holistic healer or nutritionist something more specific for your individuality.

———

Carbogenic Type Mineral Needs

Apply this mineral data to the diet following the Muscle type descriptions.

Excessive Foods:

- *Carbon (simple carbohydrates)*
- *Sodium (salted, junk)*
- *Nitrogen (beef)*

Deficient Foods:

- *Calcium*
- *Sodium (unsalted)*
- *Potassium*
- *Nitrogen (non-beef, vegetable)*
- *Magnesium*

These deficient nutrients are common deficiencies in your type, and predispose you to ill-health.
If ill, use these lists with your daily food intake.
If not ill, eat from the food lists 3-4 days weekly for health maintenance.
All food lists are in descending order of concentration and value to you; choose servings of foods in the upper half of each list first!
One serving is ½ cup.

Carbogenic Excessive Foods -

Carbon, particularly simple carbohydrates, may be excessive in your type causing ill-health, and fat production. It is excessive in all people who become fat or obese, and is in every cell of the body as the basis of life.

Sodium from salted junk foods is excessive in your tissues. To preserve your health and weight control you should avoid junk foods and fulfill your sodium needs from the food list without using the salt shaker. (Note that salt craving is a sign of exhausted under-active adrenal glands requiring nutritional treatment.)

Nitrogen from red meat is excessive in your diet (if eaten more than once weekly), and is a major cause of your acidity and illnesses; poultry, fish and eggs should be taken about four days weekly, with vegetarian proteins on other days (legumes, seeds, nuts and pasta).

———

Deficient Foods -

In illness or disease, it is important to correct these mineral deficiencies.

Calcium is often deficient. It is highly concen-trated in bones, joints, muscles, nerves, heart, teeth, and gums; if you have an illness or disease in any of these tissues calcium supplementation is invariably important. You thrive on dairy foods

Sodium, when naturally occurring in foods, is deficient in your type, and helps prevent arthritis.

Potassium may be deficient in your type. It is concentrated in and vital to the health of your muscles, heart, brain and all cells. If you are ill or diseased, potassium foods and supplements may help your healing.

Nitrogen from vegetable sources may be deficient (see above notes).

Magnesium is often deficient in your type, and is particularly important for your heart and digestive function.

———

Minimize

Excessive Mineral Foods

Carbon, Sodium (salted): *0-2 servings/<u>week</u> Simple carbohydrates, grains, breads, sweet fruits, sugars, fats, salt, all fast foods, packaged foods, canned and frozen foods, preserved meats (cured, smoked, canned), sauces (soy, barbecue, catsup etc.), chips (potato, corn, etc.), dill pickles, sauerkraut, bouillon cubes, peanut butter, salted nuts, crackers, canned or packaged soups, processed cheeses, commercial salad dressings, meat tenderizers.*
[And dump the salt-shaker!]

Note: If you must eat anything on the above list, keep it down to ½ cup, 0-2 times weekly!

Nitrogen (beef): *0-1 times/week*

Beef and red meats

Avoid <u>*simple*</u> *carbohydrates: white and brown sugars, high fructose corn syrup, honey, maple syrup, molasses, jellies, candy, ice cream, sodas.*

Eat <u>*complex*</u> *carbohydrates: yams, potatoes, squash, pumpkin, corn, lentils, peas, beans, green vegetables, grains (and foods made from them).*

Eat
Deficient Mineral Foods

Calcium: *1-2 servings/day*

Kelp, Swiss and cheddar cheese, turnip greens, almonds, brewer's yeast, parsley, corn tortillas, dandelion greens, Brazil nuts, watercress, tofu, dried figs, buttermilk, sunflower seeds, yogurt, milk products, ripe olives, broccoli, cottage cheese.

Also Milk: 1-2 glasses/day
Low-fat or non-fat milk, bone broths, and soups invigorate and help your healing.

Potassium, Sodium (non-junk):
1-2 servings/day

Kelp, olives, cheddar cheese, scallops, cottage cheese, dulse, blackstrap molasses, brewer's yeast, rice, gizzard, lentils, almonds, Swiss chard, beets and greens, wheat, sunflower seeds, almonds, parsley, un-hulled sesame seeds.

<u>Eat</u>
Deficient Mineral Foods

Nitrogen (vegetable and non-red meat):

Legumes, peas, cabbage, black-eyed peas, seeds, most nuts, pasta, spirulina, oranges, potatoes, soybean —as desired
Poultry, fish, eggs —2-4 days weekly

Magnesium: *1-2 servings/day*

Brewer's yeast, seeds (pumpkin, squash, sunflower, sesame), kelp, buckwheat, dulse, millet, tofu, beet greens, coconut, rye.

Note: Eat any healthy foods you desire, but be sure to include the type foods in your daily choices.

Carbogenic Nutritional Supplements

- **Multi-Vitamins** —
  [All supplements with food]
  2 capsules/ day

- **Calcium** —
  600 mg/ twice daily

- **Potassium** —
  99 mg/ day with food
  [A multi-vitamin-mineral product containing the above nutrients is appropriate.]

- **Herbs** —
  Brain detox – Chickweed or Valerian Rt.
  Organ detox – Echinacea Rt or Red Clover
  (One capsule, twice daily for one month; then one, three times weekly.)

- **Lecithin** —
  About 1,300 mg/ three times weekly

- **Evening Primrose or Flaxseed Oil**
  1 soft-gel/ day

Note: Take these supplements if you have ill-health. If in good health, take them at least 3-4 days weekly.

Important Carbogenic Health Concerns

Eating simple sugars and carbohydrates make you sick: be sure to eat a moderate protein and low simple carbohydrate diet for health and weight-control (high-protein diets are unhealthy for you). Your genetics require the *Muscle* type Food Guide, and any flesh cravings are normal and healthy for you. After about age 40-45, as your metabolism slows, you need about 3-4 flesh days weekly and vegetarian meals on other days. When ill you are often 'starch and sugar poisoned'. Other body types handle white sugar products tolerably well, but in *carbogenics and carboferics*, excessive white sugar and corn syrup intake contributes strongly to your diseases and fat accumulation.

▶ *Calcium, dairy foods, low or non-fat milk, bone broths, and soups are healing for you. You need a moderate flesh intake along with calcium and magnesium foods and supplements.*

Carbogenic Food Guide

Aim for -
50% Proteins, complex carbohydrates
50% Fruits, salads, vegetables
and
50% Raw food diet
50% Cooked foods

Eat dairy foods
Lose the salt shaker

Follow the Mineral Food recommendations.
Take the recommended supplements.

* * *

Carbogenic Weight Loss

A *carboferic* Fat type, if present, causes fat accumulation with aging. Losing weight depends upon you following the type instructions, summarized in this section.

- *Stop* eating carbon, sodium foods (see list)
- *Protein* drink, about 25-30 grams daily
- *Eat* your body type deficient mineral foods daily
- *Follow* your *Carbogenic Factors* (as above)
- *Exercise*: your body type requires moderate to intense daily exercise

- *Simple sugars*: stop all white table sugar and high-fructose corn syrup and drinks containing these sugars
- *Mental balance and positive thinking:* you may be mentally stressed by everyday life, which causes adrenal hypoglycemia, low blood sugar; you need to take these supplements: *calcium/magnesium*, two capsules, and *chamomile,* two capsules, both with food
- *Adrenal Hypoglycemia:* this hormonal imbalance stops fat loss, and usually initiates more fat production, so it is vital to deal with this problem: take *pantothenic acid,* 500 mg/twice daily with food
- *Pancreatic Hypoglycemia:* as above, this hormonal imbalance causes sugar craving and you need: *Fo-ti herb,* two capsules, twice daily with food
- *Calories:* As with any dietary approach, calories in. must be *less than* calories out! Most markets sell a calorie booklet; note your daily intake and, in most instances, keep it under about 1500 calories/day

Note that some of you overindulge in milk; although it is healing for you I have known several men who craved calcium so much that they drank 3-4 quarts of milk daily ending up with kidney stones and other hardening diseases.

———

Muscle Types
General Food Guide

(Carnivores)

Important Note

――――

The Food Guide addresses the <u>Acid-Alkaline</u> aspect of your food intake, along with the <u>Type Mineral</u> factor presented throughout this book. It does <u>not</u> necessarily address calories or other dietary factors that may be pertinent to your personal health needs whether medical or appropriate for some other dietary need. So use your common sense and just include the factors described here with whatever healthy dietary choices you usually make.

For other nutrient information, consult with nutritional books or with holistic nutritional doctors. In this regard, I particularly recommend the advice of Andrew Weil, M.D.

――――

Muscle Types
General Food Guide

(Not for the Nitropheric Type)

This chapter presents a general Food Guide, upon which you superimpose the nutritional information from your type chapter. As a Muscle body type your genetics require flesh foods.

———

Meat/Flesh Intake

Most muscle types should limit red meat to once or less weekly, while eggs, lamb, fish, or poultry are excellent in moderation. If ill or diseased, be sure to eat daily, one or two servings from each *deficient minerals* list. If not ill, eat them at least three times weekly for health maintenance. If this diet is similar to your present diet, but healing is sluggish, then:

- Decrease your carbohydrate and protein intake by about one-third
- Increase your fruit, salad, and vegetable intake by about one-third
- Consult with a holistic doctor, preferably one versed in nutritional and emotional evaluation

———

Over-Acid or Over-Alkaline?

Just as a log of wood burned in your fireplace leaves a mineral-ash, food ash refers to the minerals remaining after metabolizing foods in your tissues:

- Fruits, vegetables *alkalinize* tissues
- Proteins, carbohydrates *acidify* tissues

Usually You Are Over-Acid Due To:

- Excessive intake of dairy foods
- Excessive intake of proteins and carbohydrates
- Deficient intake of fruits, salads and vegetables
- Accumulated metabolic waste-acids (from years of eating excessive acid-ash foods, meats and carbohydrates, and from lack of exercise)
- You need to estimate the ratio of foods eaten. Generally, eat the following *approximate* ratios for your health:

50% <u>Alkaline-ash</u> foods *(fruits, salads, vegetables)*

50% <u>Acid-ash</u> foods *(complex carbohydrates like starches, grains, cereals, breads, flour products; and proteins)*

Approximate your food ratios. On any particular day, it does not matter if one meal is mostly alkaline, and another mostly acid—just try to balance it out for the day! If you get it wrong, try again tomorrow. It is a subjective call that you make, and it is what you do over weeks, months, or years that make the difference—not on any one or two days.

———

Note - If Vegetarian

As a general indication, if you follow a vegetarian diet substitute vegetable sources of protein for the any flesh in the food guide. Note that contrary to most alkaline-ash vegetarian diets you need something different:

*You need an **acid-ash** vegetarian diet high in complex carbohydrates and vegetable proteins.*

Because of your high need for protein, you usually require a vegetable powdered protein supplement in juice (about 25-30 grams daily).

———

Important

- Minimize white sugar and alcohol intake.
- If desired, interchange lunches for dinners.

- Never eat foods you are allergic to, no matter what I recommend; if allergic, or suspect a food allergy, eliminate it and substitute from your type mineral lists.
- Eat the right foods 80-90% of the time and the Food Guide will work for you; unlike some types you do not have to live out of a health food store (although such foods are healthier for you).

▶ *Omit eating the excessive minerals in your type chapter, and be sure to eat one or two servings from the deficient list daily.*

Finally, in addition to your body type needs, other holistic healing matters also need your attention. I strongly suggest that you refer to my web site and earlier books for that information: *DrStenbeck.net*

———

Acid/Alkaline Genetics Chart

The following chart reflects each Muscle Type and its acid or alkaline-ash food needs. These ratios change if you are unhealthy or over age 45-50. Refer back to your body type and review the *Acid/alkaline* instructions.

———

Acid/Alkaline Genetics, Dietary-Ash, and Raw Food Needs

This chart shows the Rocine types, their acid or alkaline food needs, and the percentage of raw foods needed for your health and healing.

- Apply your Type Minerals to the Food Guide

Type	Acid/Alkaline Genetics	% Food-Ash Needed	% Raw Food Needed
Calciferic	Alkaline	70% acid	30
Carbogenic	Alkaline	50-50	50
Desmogenic	Alkaline	70% acid	50
Eldic	Intermediate	50-50	50
Medeic	Intermediate	50-50	50
Myogenic	Intermediate	50-50	50
Nervimotive	Alkaline	70% acid	50
Nitropheric	Acid	70% <u>alkaline</u>	70
Pallinomic	Alkaline	50-50	30

The above percentages vary depending on aging and the health of individual types.

Muscle Types General Food Guide
Breakfast

[Superimpose the nutritional information from your

EGGS* *(1-2) with lettuce, tomato, or salad, whole grain toast; (add bacon or sausage 1-3 times weekly if desired)*
— 2-4 times/week; or

FRUIT *fresh salad, and protein (yogurt, milk, cheeses, seeds, nuts)*
—1-3 times/week; or

CEREALS, *with fruit, seeds, nuts*
—2-5 times/week; or

OTHER *choices*
— 0-1 times weekly

Daily liquids:
Pure water, citrus, vegetable juices, soups, other —as desired
Coffee, teas —0-2 cups

[Include selections from your type mineral needs everyday.]

Lunch

SALADS, mixed green, protein (poultry, fish, egg, cheese, seeds or nuts, etc.), whole grain breads
[Dressing: olive oil/ vinegar; low-fat, low-cal dressings]
— 2-4 times/ week; or

SANDWICH, whole grains with a protein (cheese, tuna, ham, etc.); and salad and/ or vegetables
— 1-4 times/ week; or

POULTRY, FISH, 3-6 oz., with a mixed green salad and/ or vegetables
—1-3 times/ week; or

OTHER choices (with salad or vegetables)
—1-2 times/ week

[Other oils permitted, but less ideal is soybean oil, a common allergen; minimize commercial dressings. Be sure to include two or more selections from your type food lists in your daily food intake. For in-between meal snacks, eat fruit or vegetables with seeds/ nuts.]

[Include selections from your type mineral needs everyday.]

Dinner

POULTRY, FISH *(4-6 oz.), with salad and/or vegetables*
—2-4 times/week; or

PASTA *with protein (chicken, etc.) with salad and/or vegetables*
— 2-4 times/week; or

VEGETARIAN *meal with salad and/or vegetables*
—1-3 times/week; or

LEAN BEEF *(4-6 oz.) with salad and/or vegetables*
— 0-1 times/week

OTHER *choices with salad and/or vegetables*
— 0-1 times/week

Desserts:
Fruits, fresh —as desired
Low-sugar, healthy desserts
— 0-3 times/wk

[Include selections from your type mineral needs everyday.]

Food Guide Notes

Steamed Vegetables —

Minerals are lost in the boiling of vegetables; steaming or wok cooking is best.

Food Combinations —

If you have a weak digestive system then eating proteins at the same meal with starches often results in indigestion, gas, or constipation.

Periodic Detox —

You tend to over-indulge in acid-ash foods (proteins and carbohydrates), and often need occasional elimination diets for tissue waste-acid removal. Have a holistic doctor or nutritionist supervise such detox (where you have an alkaline-ash diet along with protein supplementation).

Minimize —

- Fatty foods
- Commercial salad dressings
- Beef, red meats, processed meats
- Coffee, white sugar, corn syrup, alcohol

Vegetarian Proteins —

You require a carnivorous diet. An exception is the *nitropheric* type who functions best with a *vegetarian* diet. The other muscle types are born to be carnivores. It is very difficult for the other muscle types to be pure vegetarians because of their strong intuitive cravings for fish, poultry, meat, or eggs. If you are vegetarian, then because of your high needs for amino acids and acid-ash foods, you should take a protein supplement of 30-40 grams/day (powdered protein in juice).

Healthy Weight —

Several of you gain weight as the ravages of age, lack of exercise and dietary excesses take their toll. By eating according to your body type, you should naturally lose excess weight. Each type also has a few individual factors that only apply to them!

You have a good ability to lose weight by following the Food Guide instructions. The most common problem I find with your weight-control is liver and kidney irritation due to food allergies, which results in extra pounds. The key is to eat non-allergic foods.

If drinking more than 3-4 cups daily of coffee or tea, you may have a hypoglycemic problem (low blood sugar), which contributes to making fat, ill-health, and delayed healing. (Refer to the earlier books for help with this healing.)

———

Appendix

Brief Extracts from
<u>The 22 Unique Body Types</u>

Appendix A

Types

(Brief extract)

Type comes from 'typus' meaning an image or impression, the study of types being called typology.

▶ *Rocine: "A combination of mental and structural features is consistently found in people of the same type."*

Rocine wrote that all types are a mixture of positive and negative qualities. He based his work on the biochemical individuality of our *mineral* absorption and utilization. Of course, all minerals are absorbed, but he postulated that different types of people *selectively* absorb certain minerals, to a greater or lesser extent, requiring specific mineral foods for their enhanced health and healing. This is the basis of his types.

▶ *The type information cannot predict what or who you will become, or how successful or not, but your type is capable of bringing a creative excellence to whatever you do in life. If your type has negative qualities that you disagree with, remember that they are only tendencies and may or may not manifest in you.*

This book enlarges on Rocine's premise (early 1900's), integrated with the later research of Herbert Sheldon, M.D., Ph.D., at Harvard University (1930's), along with my fifty years of observations and experience with this subject.

Comparing your shared physical (and sometimes psychological) descriptions with the Celebrity Lists further assists the identification of your type. It is not that you will look exactly like, or be a twin to, any particular celebrity. Look closely at a celebrity's features: face, profile, height, weight, head, etc. If you know something about their talents, beliefs, success and failure spheres, health and weight challenges, attitudes and behaviors, etc., then you get clues as to what your type may be.

———

Understanding Types and Sub-Types

Each of us has a clearly discernible dominant type. Visualize the celebrity examples from movies, politics, sports, the arts and public life, and try to identify with their physical features. Look for similar features, remembering that you will not recognize all attributes in yourself. You are not looking for your twin!

The sub-type issue is the main reason people of the same major type can look so different. Remember that a type description does not characterize you exactly, but depicts your individual variant of a type.

▶ *The type questionnaire pinpoints the major features of that type: if the celebrity examples are unhelpful, you may be an unusual variant (in which case ignore the celebrity issue and give yourself 7 points on Question 1).*

———

Minerals
(Brief Extract)

Minerals are essential life nutrients that accelerate enzyme and chemical reactions and provide a basis for your body typing. Although found in all tissues, different minerals tend to be concentrated in certain organs, their presence or absence contributing to the healing of such tissues; e.g., zinc accelerates prostate healing; calcium and manganese promote bone, joint and connective tissue healing.

Specific foods nurture each type, some people needing meats for their health others needing a vegetarian diet. A high potassium diet nurtures one person, while another needs high sulfur, calcium, zinc, or another mineral.

Mineral Digestion and Absorption

Compared to vitamins, minerals are *difficult* to digest, absorb, and utilize. In people with strong digestive systems, this aspect may not be important. The following factors should be in place for optimal mineral metabolism:
1. Stomach Hydrochloric Acid Production
2. Parathyroid Hormone Balance
3. Organ Toxic Metal and Chemical Removal
   [See details in The 22 Unique Body Types.]

———

Total Body Healing

Note that from a holistic healing perspective, in addition to minerals and type information, the following healing factors are necessary:

> *Nutrient Balance*
> *Mental Balance*
> *Emotional Balance*
> *Spiritual Balance*
> *Detoxifying Integrity*

The above factors are all important to your total healing especially if you are interested in self-healing (see my earlier books).

———

Appendix B

Researchers

(Brief extract)

The predominant workers in this area of human individuality from around 1880's to the 1960's are Herbert Sheldon, M.D., Ph.D., Roger Williams, Ph.D., and Victor Rocine, D.Sc.

Much information on Sheldon's research exists on-line and in medical psychology libraries; for interested readers there are other lines of research published in the last century. This present book is primarily about Rocine's body types.

Herbert Sheldon M.D., Ph.D.

In contrast to Rocine, Sheldon at Harvard University in the 1930's was trained in the scientific method and did painstaking research and publishing on human individuality. In comparing his findings with Rocine's work, a direct putative correlation is visible.

Roger J. Williams, Ph.D.

Another significant researcher in human individuality is the renowned scientist and biochemist, Roger J. Williams. He demonstrated that different people have varying levels of nutrients, enzymes, and other metabolic chemicals in their bloodstreams.

▶ *Williams's research firmly expands on the premise of individual nutritional needs in human beings. If interested in his research, I highly recommend his book Biochemial Individuality.*

Victor Rocine, D.Sc.

Note that when a negative feature is indicated, say neurotic tendencies, all members of the type are <u>not</u> that way; it is a type tendency reported by Rocine.

Rocine studied type-related diseases finding links between mineral and dietary factors with individual types and their diseases. In each body type, one or more dominant minerals are preferentially absorbed and utilized over other minerals.

He recognized discrete body types from their physical appearance finding genetically based mineral dominance to be the determining feature. He also correlated their physical features with psychological characteristics.

———

Appendix C

Genetics, Types, and Diet
(Brief extract)

This section deals with how nervous system genetics helps determine your eating choices for health: you are either born to be a predominant meat eater, a partial or complete vegetarian, or something between the two. The genetic factor determining this dietary aspect is the *sympathetic and parasympathetic* components of your central nervous system. This represents a basic factor in eating for health.

This chapter helps you understand your dietary inheritance, although instinctively, you may already have arrived there:

- If born **sympathetic** dominant you are *genetically acid*, desiring a predominantly *vegetarian* diet for your health (about 70% fruit, salad, vegetables to 30% proteins and carbohydrates).

- If born **parasympathetic** dominant you are *genetically alkaline*, desiring a predominantly *carnivorous* diet for your health (about 70% proteins, carbohydrates to 30% fruits, salads, vegetables). Few of you ever choose to become vegetarian because of the difficulty in satisfying your protein needs without meats.

- If born *intermediate* dominant you may eat food groups with little concern for the acid/alkaline factor. However, after age 40, you need a semi-vegetarian diet for healthy eating.

Chart: Relative Nervous System Dominance

In the following Chart, if you relate to many of the symptoms on one side you probably have that nervous system dominance; relating to both sides indicates *Intermediate* dominance.

If Vegetarian (Over-acid)
Eat: 70% fruits, salads, vegetables
And 30% proteins, carbohydrates

If Carnivore (Over-alkaline)
Eat 70% proteins, carbohydrates
And 30% fruits, salads, vegetables

If Intermediate
Eat 50:50 of acid and alkaline-ash foods

Make an *approximate* estimate of your daily acid and alkaline food intake (such ratios varying from type to type).

Symptoms of Relative Genetic Dominance

Vegetarians (Over-acid)	Carnivores (Over-alkaline)
Sympathetic Dominance	Parasympathetic Dominance
little or no flesh desire	desire flesh
easily constipated	rarely constipated
slow digestion	fast digestion
easily dehydrated	not dehydrated
strong thirst	low thirst
pale face	flushed face
high pulse after food	slow pulse after food
easy gag reflex	slow gag reflex
cool dry skin	moist warm skin
nervous stomach	calm stomach
little eyelid blinking	much blinking
nervous tendency	mostly calm
slower healing	faster healing
low oxygen-uptake	good oxygen-uptake
easily breathless	seldom breathless
insomnia common	sleep easier
few muscle cramps	some night cramps
calcium deposits rare	get calcium deposits

Appendix D

Help Identifying your Body Type with Dr. Stenbeck

If you desire help in identifying your body type, follow these instructions, and answer the questionnaire. For further information and fees, send me an email from page one of the website:

DrStenbeck.net

First name: _____

Country of birth: _____

Upload photos and send to the above website:

■ Head and shoulders: front and side views

■ Full body: front and side views

■ Also 1-2 teenage views

■ If possible, casual photos of mother, father, siblings

MY TYPE CLASS MAY BE: _____

(Thin, Muscle, or Fat)

AGE   -   _____

HEIGHT   -   _____ feet/inches

MY WEIGHT -   _____ pounds

- Heaviest at age: _____

    - Lightest as adult: _____

    - Estimate age 15: _____

VISION - Excellent Average   Poor:

HAIR - Natural color: _____

    - Thin/thick? _____

    - balding? _____

SKIN - Quality: _____

    - History of acne, boils, other:

_____

_____

TEETH -   Strong Weak   Dentures

 - Cavity history: Many   Moderate Few

MUSCLES - Strong Average Weak

    Sports played _____

JOINTS -   Strong Average Weak

HEALTH - Childhood diseases?

_____

_____

    - Adult diseases?

_____

AVERAGE DIET

- Beef _____ (times/week)

- Poultry _____ (times/week)

- Fish _____ (times/week)

- Eggs _____ (times/week)

- Water _____ (glasses/day):

- Vegetarian? Vegan? _____

- Other? _____

- Did your childhood diet differ? _____

The above will help me know who you are! I will send you a follow-up questionnaire for further help in identifying your body type.

Appendix E

On-line Health Consultation with Dr. Stenbeck

For further information, or to comment on this book, or to receive a response on any health issue from a holistic viewpoint, send an email inquiry from page one of my website:

DrStenbeck.net

Following that, I will suggest further healing needs, which we may pursue with an on-line consult.

———

Appendix F

Notes

See my book *The 22 Unique Body Types,* available at the usual online source, for further information and details on all of the 22 Types. The Appendix in that book has further information about:

Mineral Functions and Food Sources

Further Reading

———

www.ingramcontent.com/pod-product-compliance
Lightning Source LLC
Chambersburg PA
CBHW062100280526
45788CB00003B/1297